Smoothie Cleanse & Healthy Detox

Moneva Amanda

Table of Content

SMOOTHIE CLEANSE & HEALTHY DETOX 1

PREFACE 6

INTRODUCTION 8

CHAPTER 1 9

    FRUIT AND GREEN SMOOTHIE RECIPES FOR WEIGHT LOSS 9

        Kale-Banana-Apple Cider Smoothie 9

        Spinach-Peach-Mango Smoothie 10

        Spinach-Apple-Ginger Smoothie 11

        Collard Greens-Berries Smoothie 13

        Dr Oz's Green Smoothie 14

        Romaine Lettuce-Apple Green Smoothie 15

        Spinach-Grapefruit Smoothie 17

        Spinach-Banana Smoothie 18

    OTHER WEIGHT LOSS SMOOTHIE RECIPE 19

        Fat Reducing Smoothie 19

CHAPTER 2 22

    THE WEIGHT LOSS MECHANISM OF SMOOTHIE 22

    FOODS FOR LOSING FAT AND BOOSTING THE METABOLISM 23

    OTHER FOODS THAT HELPS YOU LOSE WEIGHT 24

CHAPTER 3 28

    DETOXIFICATION 28

        Marijuana Detoxification and Drinks 28

    MOST POPULAR CLEANSING DRINKS 30

        Clear Choice 30

        The Best Detox Cleansing Drink 30

        Toxin Rid 31

        One-Shot Focus 31

        Rescue Cleansing Blueberry Ice 31

        Stinger 32

CHAPTER 4 34

HOMEMADE DETOX DRINKS 34
- *Lemon Juice* 35
- *Vinegar* 35
- *Cranberry Juice* 36

ARE CLEANSING WINES RESULTIVE? 37

CHAPTER 5 39

BEST DETOX DRINK FOR A DRUG TEST 39
WHAT FOODS TO CONSUME THROUGHOUT A DRUG OR ALCOHOL DETOX 42
FOODS TO AVOID DURING DETOX 46

CHAPTER 6 48

BEST FRUITS SMOOTHIES FOR MELTING BELLY FAT 48
- *Refreshing Raspberry Cream Smoothie* 51

CHAPTER 7 53

BREAKFAST SMOOTHIES FOR FLAT BELLY 53

CHAPTER 8 65

SMOOTHIES FOR HEALTHY DIGESTION 65
- *Steps to make Smoothies Better to Digest* 65

HEALTHY DIGESTIVE SYSTEM SMOOTHIES 66
- *Mango & Turmeric Healthy Digestive system Smoothie* 67
- *Blueberry & Beet Healthy Digestive System Smoothie* 69
- *Pineapple & Kale Healthy Digestive system Smoothie* 71

CHAPTER 9 73

GREEN SMOOTHIES THAT HEAL THE GUT & INCREASE ENERGY 73
- *Belly Cleanser Green Smoothie* 73
- *Cheery Cherry Detoxification Smoothie* 74
- *Pineapple Ginger Green Detox Smoothie* 76
- *Orange Cleansing Drink* 77
- *Strawberry Detoxification Green Monster Smoothie* 78
- *Cleansing Blueberry Monster Smoothie* 79

Basic Kale Detoxification Juice *80*

CHAPTER 9 .... **82**

SMOOTHIES FOR RADIANT SKIN 82

CHAPTER 10 .... **96**

SMOOTHIES FOR WEIGHT LOSS AND BODY DETOX 96

Copyright © 2021 by Moneva Amanda

All rights reserved. No part of this publication may be reproduced, distributed, or transmitted in any form or by any means, including photocopying, recording, or other E or mechanical methods, without the prior written permission of the publisher, except in the case of brief quotations embodied in critical reviews and certain other non-commercial uses permitted by copyright law.

ISBN: 978-1-63750-311-9

Preface

Are you looking for a clean and healthy way to "reset" your body? Are you looking for fast and simple ways to lose weight? If so, this is going to be the most valuable information you will ever receive.

Are you ready to take the health and energy levels of an elite athlete and fold them into your daily routine? If so, this book is for you. It contains delicious and easy-to-prepare juices and smoothies recipes. Each recipe was created by a respected expert in the field of healthy living and contains all the important details you need to create your very own superfood powerhouse. You'll also learn the amazing benefits of fresh fruit and vegetable juices and blends as part of a cleansing diet to help flush out toxins from your body.

Don't let the name fool you. These recipes are not just for weight loss. They are also great for building lean muscle mass... improving your skin... and much, much more!

Most people who follow these juice and smoothie recipes lose 1 to 2 pounds per day. These simple and easy-to-prepare recipes will put the "pump" back into your step and leave you feeling re-energized.

Introduction

Would you like to lose weight naturally? You might need to begin detoxification and taking in some healthy smoothies now. I resolved my being overweight by consuming healthy fruits and veggie smoothie with quality recipes for weight loss.

I've probably attempted all the dietary plan fads on the market, but without any real results. I had been close to quitting when a friend launched me to green smoothies and other healthy smoothies as well as exercise and healthy living. I've seen noticeable leads as soon as two weeks.

To help overweight people and healthy living enthusiasts, here are healthy smoothies with tested recipes that you can check at home.

Chapter 1
Fruit and Green Smoothie Recipes For Weight Loss
Kale-Banana-Apple Cider Smoothie

This green smoothie combines **_Kale with Banana and apple cider_** to provide powerful _detoxifying benefits_. The trick ingredient of the formula is _apple cider_. It gives that juicy green apple flavor. A dash of _cinnamon_ is also added to bring spice to the complete concoction.

The **_Banana_** in this recipe works as the bottom fruit giving that thick texture to your smoothie. The **_Kale_** is the leafy green that offers various nutrition like _magnesium, folate, and dietary fiber_. Finally, **_Apple cider_** provides weight loss benefits and alleviation towards symptoms of diabetes.

To start this smoothie formula, prepare these substances:

- Half of a banana.
- 1 cup of _Kale_, without stems.
- 1/2 cup Apple cider.
- 1/2 cup water.

- A dash of cinnamon.

Put all ingredients, aside from the cinnamon, in a blender and combine until clean. If the constituent is too thick, add water. If the structure is too slim, add a banana. When already smooth, add the cinnamon and put it into a cup to serve.

Spinach-Peach-Mango Smoothie

This green smoothie combines **_spinach_** with many sweet fruits, like **_bananas, peaches, and mango_**. If you're not a spinach lover, this smoothie is a superb way to take this leafy green as its flavor is masked well with the fruits. Nevertheless, you can't face concealing the outstanding nutrition of spinach.

***Spinach** has anti-inflammatory benefits as well as anti-cancer properties.* Additionally, it is an excellent way to obtain nutritional *vitamins A, C, and E*. In the meantime, peaches contain bioactive properties that have demonstrated characteristics in fighting weight problems.

For this formula, you will need a blender and these substances:

- 1 frozen banana.
- 1/4 cup peaches.
- 1/4 cup frozen mango.
- A small quantity of spinach.
- Water.

Blend all elements in a blender until even. Pour the completed smoothie in a cup or mason jar. Enjoy while still cold.

Spinach-Apple-Ginger Smoothie

Spinach and *apple* make a great smoothie combo. This combo is manufactured extra spicy with the help of *ginger*. Rather than using water, you may use coconut water to improve the nutrition. *Cucumber* provides that refreshing flavor into the blend with fewer calorie consumption to boot.

Regarding **Dr. Axe**, cucumber can help you lose weight by quenching your thirst and limit your desire to consume credited to dehydration. *Ginger* also provides that same appetite retardant result. A lot more than the weight loss benefits offered by these substances, they clear your skin layer from lines, wrinkles, and other blemishes.

Apart from a blender and a mason jar, here will be the things that you'll need:

- 1 cup spinach, chopped
- 1 apple, cored and diced
- 1 cucumber
- 2 cups of coconut water
- A thumb-sized ginger
- A small quantity of parsley

Add all ingredients in a blender until steady. Serve in a mason jar and drink during breakfast for the best results.

Have you loved pursuing these healthy fruits and veggie smoothie dishes for weight loss?

This list is essential if you ask me since it may help lose weight relatively. Plus, consuming these smoothies improves general health.

Collard Greens-Berries Smoothie

This smoothie recipe, adapted from Lean Secrets, combines **_collard greens_** with **_berries_** and **_wheatgrass_** *to make a highly resulting weight loss drink.* Collard greens are perfect for weight loss because they contain surprisingly low-calorie consumption. In addition, this dark leafy green can be considered a great way to obtain nutritional ***vitamins A, C, and B6.***

The wheat lawn is rich with proteins; its grassy flavor can be masked with the sweetness of *berries. Macca natural powder gives a power increase, while coconut water can offer antioxidant power.*

Listed below are the ingredients of the *grassy smoothie recipe*:

- 2 cups of coconut water.
- 3 cups of frozen berries.
- 1 cup collard greens.
- 1 cup wheatgrass.
- 1 tablespoon of maca powder.
- Stevia

To create this formula, just blend the ingredients entirely in a blender for approximately one minute or until it gets to your desired regularity. From then on, you can transfer the completed smoothie into a cup and drink in an empty belly for better nutritional absorption.

Dr Oz's Green Smoothie

Dr Oz shares his favorite green drink to begin your early morning right. Substitute your regular early morning drink with this low-calorie drink, and you're on the right course of your bodyweight loss program. *Coupled with spinach and apples, you can get a fibre-rich drink to begin your day.*

The <u>orange, pineapple, lime, and lemon</u> are rich in **Vitamin C** *to strengthen your disease-fighting capability.* <u>Cucumber</u> *consists of high degrees of* **B** *nutritional vitamins to relieve stress and drive back the damaging ramifications of stress.*

<u>Celery</u> *is a superb source of* **vitamin K** *to avoid excessive blood loss. At the same time,* <u>Carrots</u> *contain* **beta-carotene** *for pores and skin and vision health.*

To produce this green smoothie, you'll need these

elements:

- 1 cup spinach
- 1/4 cup cucumber
- 3/4 cup parsley, chopped
- 1/2 glass mint, chopped
- 1/4 mind of celery
- 1 apple
- 1/4 of each- orange, lime, lemon, and pineapple
- 2 carrots, peeled

In a blender, blend all ingredients. If you discover the combination is too thick for your choice, add drinking water. Pour the completed smoothie in a mason jar or any cup of your choice and serve. Enjoy while still chilly.

Romaine Lettuce-Apple Green Smoothie

Clinical nutritionist *Kimberly Snyder* recommends this wonderful *smoothie recipe for energy boost, weight loss, and excellent skin.* In addition, **Romaine lettuce** *is an excellent source of nutritional vitamins A, K, and iron.* You'll get more *vitamin A* from a mind of *romaine lettuce* than a big carrot.

The *apple and pear* in this recipe give a weight loss benefit as they fulfill your craving for food for a small number of calories. *Relating to a 2003 research, regular intake of **pears** and **apples** may donate to weight loss.* To thicken the persistence of the smoothie, I added one freezing *Banana*.

Eager to begin this recipe? Listed below are ingredients you'll need:

- 1 head romaine lettuce, chopped.
- 3/4 pound spinach.
- 3 celery stalks.
- 1 apple, cored, and diced.
- 1 pear, cored, and diced.
- 1 frozen banana.
- Half of a lemon, juiced

Inside a blender, add water and *romaine lettuce*. Mix until roughly combined, then add all of those other ingredients. Mix until fine, and serve in a mason jar or large cup. Drink this ideally each day to get the best results.

Spinach-Grapefruit Smoothie

Another Refreshing smoothie mixture includes *spinach, grapefruit, and Banana*. The *grapefruit* offers a tart taste as the *Banana* amounts it using its natural sweetness. Apart from their delectable tastes, they're filled with essential nutrition, like *vitamin A, potassium, and vitamin C.*

Grapefruits have a negligible quantity of calorie consumption, but they're rich in nutritional *vitamins A and C*; Also, they provide a little increase to your weight loss diet.

Listed below are the things that you require to get ready:

- 1 grapefruit, peeled and deseeded.
- 1 apple, cored and peeled.
- 2 cups spinach.
- 1 frozen banana.
- Almond milk.
- Ice cubes

Within a blender, put all the ingredients and combine them until it gets to your desired consistency. Be sure you add more ice if too slim, which will offer you a shake-like uniformity. You can even add more Bananas if you discover the blend is too blanded for your flavor.

Spinach-Banana Smoothie

This smoothie recipe is easy to do because all you'll need are four ingredients; **Coconut milk, Yoghurt, Banana,** and **Spinach**. They form a low-calorie drink collectively, which can enhance your energy and make your skin layer glow. In addition, *consuming this smoothie every day will limit your urges for sweet snack foods; hence, you lose pounds on the way.*

As you know, *spinach* is saturated in nutritional *vitamins K, A, and C. Bananas* support weight loss by causing you to feel full for an extended period, hence less calorie consumption. To miss the use of ice, you may use a frozen banana in the smoothie. You have to learn how to squeeze Banana for smoothies

Listed below are the things that you'll need:

- 1 cup of organic coconut milk.

- 6 ounces of non-fat Greek yogurt.

- 1 frozen banana.

- 2 cups spinach, chopped.

In a blender, put all ingredients and mix well. Add a little water if you discover the regularity is too dense for your liking. Serve in a mason jar or cup of your choice.

Other Weight Loss Smoothie Recipe

This weight loss smoothie is a bit harder than our most popular smoothie recipe, but we believe it can help you observe results quicker when coupled with an incredible exercise goal. We wish you give it a go and love the results just as much as we do. Happy mixing!

Fat Reducing Smoothie

Description

Make fat weep with the addition of this thick reducing smoothie into your entire day. The 100% natural ingredients are combined jointly to help increase your metabolism and get rid of fat in a single delicious weight loss smoothie.

Ingredients

- 2 cups spinach
- 1/4 cup fresh mint leaves.
- 2 stalks celery (chopped).
- 1 cup brewed green tea extract (cooled).
- 1 large grapefruit (peeled and seeded).
- 2 cups of pineapple chunks (frozen).
- 1/2 large avocado.
- 1/8 teaspoon floor cayenne pepper (optional)

Instructions

- Place spinach, mint, celery, and green tea extract into a blender.
- Puree until fine.
- Add staying ingredients (grapefruit, pineapple, avocado, and cayenne pepper).
- Blend again.

You can serve and take your smoothie.

Chapter 2
The Weight Loss Mechanism of Smoothie

Why Smoothies Assist You to Lose Weight

For the majority of us, there's an equilibrium between your good stuff and the not-so-good things. (*I'm speaking of French fries with my veggie burger.*) My point is, it's always hard to eat healthily. Which explains why I sponsor a quarterly cleanse using green smoothies every day. I offer you an organized meal intending to concentrate on eating the foodstuffs that will assist us to enjoy the best.

You will find special occasions whenever we want to indulge; it's hard to consume healthy at all times, especially when traveling. You understand the drill. We do our best, but we don't have the confidence to occasionally prepare ourselves to enjoy a delicacy.

I'm a large proponent of eating healthy whenever you can and taking part in a regular workout routine. That appears different for all those with our assorted passions, schedules, time constraints, and lifestyles. There's nothing at all that will assist or increase your metabolism more than working out and building your muscle.

More muscle means more fat-burning capabilities. So when we're discussing how to improve metabolism, exercise will go together with healthy eating. In addition, particular foods with fat-burning and metabolism-boosting abilities and adding them into your daily diet can help magnify weight-loss attempts. I'm an enormous smoothie lover, especially when I use 100% natural ingredients to change it into a weight loss smoothie.

Foods for Losing Fat and Boosting The Metabolism

The body needs the proper energy to maintain the needs of day-to-day activities. Therefore, it's essential to know the quantity and quality of calories we consume, particularly if we're attempting to lose weight, gain muscle, or improve our performance.

What does this mean? It means that we have to tick off several containers: healthy fat, protein, complicated carbs, minerals and vitamins, and a mixture of all the above. A fat-reducing smoothie, which I'll demonstrate steps to make below, will meet your need along the way!

A protein bar may be saturated in calories and filled with nutrition, but it won't fill you up just as a bowl of salmon, brownish grain, and steamed vegetables will. Still, a high-quality (ideally homemade) protein pub can provide you with the energy you will need to power through a good workout or get over one.

Other Foods that helps you Lose Weight

Once I lose weight, I love to get a tone too. Therefore I exercise. So when we exercise (*this includes cardio, endurance operation, lifting weights, and things such as Mix Fit), we* burn off calorie consumption. Still, if our muscles need nourishment, we'll go for an easy and straightforward source first, and that's not heading to be surplus fat.

Give the body energy *(i.e. high-quality calorie consumption)* to power it through a good workout. The workout will subsequently help build more muscle, which burns up more calorie consumption (*i.e. fat*) all of those other times. Observe how perfectly that works? It's a sweet thing!

There are some foods you can mix into a weight loss smoothie if you're trying to improve your metabolism and get rid of fat:

1. ***Nut products*** - whole, preferably natural and unblanched (*almonds, walnuts, pecans); good body fat and proteins; almonds contain L-arginine (an amino acidity*), whenever used pre-workout, can help your body burn up more fat.

2. ***Eggs*** - saturated in proteins which helps increase metabolism; your body digests the proteins and uses the excess fat and calories for fuel.

3. ***Berries*** - lower in sugar but sweet, saturated in fibre, saturated in antioxidants; helps get rid of fat; can help improve blood circulation.

4. ***Apple cider vinegar*** - the acetic acidity in **ACV** supports blood sugar.

5. ***Grapefruit*** -high in phytochemicals that stimulate the creation of the hormone adiponectin, which helps your body breakdown fat.

6. *Green and white tea* - caffeine in tea provides a natural increase in energy antioxidants in tea which can help accelerate fat-burning by aiding the liver organ in converting body fat to energy.

7. *Chilli peppers* - capsaicin, the substance within pepper aids your body in converting food to energy and belly weight loss, also works as an all-natural hunger suppressant.

8. *Spinach + other leafy greens* - chock filled with minerals and vitamins and fiber.

9. *Whole grains* - like oats and dark brown rice; high dietary fiber; slow-burning to keep you fuller for much longer and fuel your body.

10. *Coconut essential oil and essential olive oil* - healthy excess fat that helps you feel satisfied when consumed; essential coconut oil is easily digested for quick energy.

11. *Avocado* - healthy extra fat, fibre, and vitamins, particularly B6 counteracts cortisol. This stress hormone plays a part in weight loss via belly fat stores.

12. *Flaxseed* - saturated in *omega-3 essential fatty acids*.

13. *Cinnamon* - polyphenols (*powerful antioxidants*) raise the metabolism and help regulate bloodstream sugar.

14. *Pears and apples* - saturated in dietary fiber plus contain pectin, which helps to maintain good health.

15. *Grapes* - high fibre and water content.

16. *Celery* - high nutritional fibre, uses more energy to break down than it offers (*i.e. detrimental calorie consumption*).

17. *Chocolates* - <u>70% + cacao content</u> is the key part; *cacao* includes high concentrations of polyphenols that drive your body to get rid of fat.

Chapter 3
Detoxification

Why People Make use of a Detox Drink

Any company gets the right to carry out an annual or biannual medication test, plus some significant corporations choose to do the assessments even more regularly to ensure their employees aren't using illicit substances/drugs. A number of the employees look for new ways to cheat the medication checks making detoxification beverages a stylish market for various manufacturers.

However, there is no detoxification drink, which has a proven result. Using any cleansing drink, both homemade and commercially produced does not assure complete detoxing or passing a medication test.

Furthermore, the efforts to bypass the medication test are both dangerous and unlawful.

Marijuana Detoxification and Drinks

Though marijuana is thought to be the safest drug that can

arrive on the drug test by some, additionally, it is the one that mostly stands between people keeping or getting the work they need. The chemical accountable for the euphoria saturated in cannabis users is named **THC**. It remains in the torso and will arrive on drug testing a lot longer than other chemicals since it is fat-soluble, meaning it gets stored among the many fatty tissues encircling different organs in the torso. Once it is resolved, it slowly starts releasing the chemical substance, rendering it detectable in the machine for longer.

To honestly detoxify your body from all traces of marijuana on your own may take up to a month. This doesn't work if one's job has a planned medication test scheduled for a week, as it's usually the case.

Detox products state to cover up the **THC** in the machine, helping to pass the test, but it is vital to keep in mind that your body must proceed through its natural process to remove the medication to bypass the machine. So basically, because one goes by a medication test utilizing a detoxification product will not mean the medicine is no more present in your body.

Most Popular Cleansing Drinks

Today, various detox beverages exist. The next is a summary of a few of the most popular drinks that claim to remove various harmful toxins before a medication test.

Clear Choice

Some people think that this is the most resulting cleansing drink that may be purchased at this time. A substantial upside is a palatable flavor that means it is easier to offer. For this to be valid, 48 hours of abstinence from cannabis must be prepared before taking in *Clear Choice,* based on the producer. The weight decides which size is required to drink.

The maker claims that *Clear Choice's sole purpose is to help pass a medication test,* so if one follows the instructions, the probability of passing is exceptionally high.

The Best Detox Cleansing Drink

Another product that states to detox your body before a urine drug test is named *the best Detox Cleansing Drink.* The product gets rid of harmful toxins from the urine, based on the manufacturer's words. However, *the only foolproof way to have clean urine is to avoid illicit chemicals.*

Toxin Rid

The product contains tablets, fibres, and liquids. The mixture of the three ingredients helps an individual detox, based on the manufacturer's words.

One-Shot Focus

One-Shot Focus is the most typical cleansing drink in addition to *Toxin Rid*. One-Shot promises to help your body eliminate nearly every solitary toxin left out after a 10-day detoxification program.

Rescue Cleansing Blueberry Ice

Rescue cleansing ice drink gets the best detoxification drink reviews for medication testing. It is well-liked because of its simple utilization, constituents, and unique taste. It is publicized as the only type of cleansing drink for medication tests that contain antioxidants. Unlike other cleansers used in detoxification drugs, which commonly take a 48-hour toxin-free window, *rescue cleansing blueberry ice* only requires a 3-hour window-pane. It requires three urinations, around 60-90 minutes, for many people to be cleansed. The cleaning result is thought to last for approximately 5 hours.

Stinger

The manufacturers of *Stinger* declare that they have the best detoxification drink for medication tests because their elements can remove the whole body toxins on the cellular level. It is available within an assortment of tastes to make it more palatable. Users should avoid harmful toxins and drugs two times before screening. Food and beverages aren't allowed within 4 hours of eating Stinger.

The flushing by the machine through frequent urination is to occur in an hour, and you can remain clean for 6 hours. Your body's peak time is thought to be toxin-free in one hour to 90 minutes after the Stinger detoxification is taken.

Remember that some substances of detox beverages may cause allergies. Also, detox beverages do not guarantee the success of passing a medication test. The legal responsibility continues to be possible if one attempts to trick the medication test.

Chapter 4
Homemade Detox Drinks

5-Day THC Detox

This five-day cleansing program is dependant on *nutrition, exercise, and vitamins*. A well-balanced diet, a lot of water, nutritional vitamins, and regular physical exercise are recommended to eliminate the **THC** from your body.

The principal focus is on avoiding **THC** from entering the bloodstream. To take action, you need to eat fatty foods and consume a lot of carbohydrates. With regards to drinks, you need to drink *espresso and tea*. These beverages are diuretics; this means they stimulate urine creation. In this manner, the **THC** will leave the system faster.

Smoothies

If you want to undergo cleansing from drugs, you need to drink smoothies with a lot of berries, spinach, avocado, and grapefruit. Many of these elements are antioxidants, which can only help to eliminate the toxins. You need to keep in brain that if one wants to move a medication test, natural remedies aren't very reliable. They only serve as yet another tool to be utilized alongside legitimate detoxification products.

Lemon Juice

Lemon juice is much less repulsive as products created explicitly for finding your way through the medication test, but it's been known to produce the desired impact. Lemon is extremely acidic, and as possible, used for cleaning purposes throughout the house, eliminating stains and it can do the same to an organism. It flushes out unwanted harmful toxins from your body, but it can require a great deal of drinking.

Although the correct hydration and healthy food are of help for your body, this still won't guarantee a passed drug test. *Avoid illicit drugs and any chemicals for non-medical purposes.*

Vinegar

Vinegar is one of the most popular home cleaning remedies. Followers of *apple cider vinegar medication detox say it can help with weight loss, blood sugar rules, and removing toxins from your body.* Despite many anecdotal success tales, little scientific proof exists to aid its performance on medications like *opioids detoxification.*

For general cleaning, the ultimate way to do apple cider vinegar alcoholic beverages detox is by using natural, unfiltered **ACV** as it still contains enzymes, nutrients, and probiotics that are advantageous for health. *Lemon juice, apple juice, cinnamon, pepper, and ginger* can be added for flavouring.

However, those who want to use vinegar as a detox cleanse drink for a medication test should be aware of the risks involved with its consumption. It gets the potential to erode teeth enamel, irritate the neck and abdomen, and interact with some medications or vitamins, including *diuretics and insulin.* To avoid this, always pour it into one glass of water rather than take it on a clear belly.

Cranberry Juice

Folks who are not massive enthusiast of produced cleansing beverages try natural cleansers. The *Cranberry juice cleansing* medication test is an excellent example. *Cranberry juice* could very well be one of the most suggested options as it pertains to finding the right detoxification drink for the medication test. Still, doctors and naturopaths only recommend it for general cleaning. It won't help your body detox from addicting substances.

Its combination of unsweetened cranberry juice and water will help get rid of the intestines, kidneys, and lymphatic system from toxins accumulated from diet and environmental effects, and may provide results within a week.

However, this detox drink for a medication test may interact with certain medications, including *cyclosporine, diclofenac, amoxicillin, cefaclor, midazolam, and more*. One main concern is that cranberries may intensify the consequences of the blood-thinning agent known as *warfarin*. People taking these medications should speak to a health care provider before using cranberry as a detoxification drink medication test.

Are Cleansing Wines Resultive?

Do detox beverages work for medication lab tests? No, they don't. Even though many think that they are excellent options for stoners searching for a magic pill when wanting to pass a bloodstream or urine test, they don't cleanse the same manner as detox medication. Hence they don't give reliable solutions.

Some manufacturers of cleansing drink medication tests even include chemicals that mask the existence of substances and their metabolites in fluids. For instance, an oxidant like *nitrite or halogen,* can destroy the **6-MAM** *metabolite of heroin* in the urine and stop it from turning up on the test. However, this system still will not help people pass a medication test, relating to experts and many other screening companies.

Cleansing wines cannot change the body's metabolism significantly enough to help people complete a medicine test. The majority are just sugary, colored water with some added nutritional vitamins and elegant design.

Chapter 5
Best Detox Drink For a Drug Test

A cleansing drink would provide you with the opportunity to complete a medication test without much hassle. They have to help anybody cleanse their bodies. This is one of the best set of detoxification drinks that you can use to be able to complete a medication test.

- *Water* - water can be viewed as the best cleansing drink available that should cleanse the body. It could be considered as an all-natural method open to detox your body. Water promotes proper Digestive system in the body by dissolving waste materials particles and harmful toxins. Then your body would take the necessary steps to flush them out generally through your digestive system. Therefore, normal water to detoxify the body wouldn't usually bring any dangerous side effect over time.

- *Lemon Juice* - Even though water alone can detoxify the body, it is best to squeeze a little lemon to it to be able to improve the results you get. You'll find an antioxidant called ***d-limonene*** within lemon in massive amounts. This antioxidant gets the potential to break down all the toxins that may be found within your liver. Alternatively, lemon consists of citric acidity, which can absorb a toxin fighting molecule called *Aluminum Hydroxide.*

- **Green Tea Extract** - Green tea extract includes an antioxidant called *polyphenol*, which includes the capability to detoxify the body. Furthermore, this antioxidant has the potential to help the body get rid of all free radicals. Then your body can modify the harm caused by cellular material as well.

- ***Orange Juice*** - Orange juice contains a lot of vitamins and minerals. Therefore, folks who are seeking to detoxify their bodies within a brief period can think of taking in orange juice. Orange juice is also called a cleansing drink due to its impressive capability to detoxify the body.

- ***Beet Juice*** - You must have found out about beet juice, but it may also be considered an excellent detox drink designed for individuals who wish to complete a medication test. The wonderful combination of vitamins and minerals that may be present in beet juice can guide you to cleanse your body by detoxifying all the antioxidants.

- ***Fruits Smoothie*** - You'll never fail with a fruit smoothie. You can find minerals, nutritional vitamins, and nutrients in large quantities within fruit smoothies. Furthermore, you'll be able to discover a massive amount of antioxidants, which will make them a perfect detoxifier. Therefore, individuals who are planning to undergo a medication test can think of taking in several fruit smoothies with no doubt on the brain.

- ***Green Juice*** - *Spinach, broccoli, and Kale* can guide you to make the best *green juices*. They are known as excellent detoxifiers as well. The dietary ingredients that are available in these juices can deliver fantastic leads to individuals when coupled with antioxidants.

What Foods to Consume Throughout a Drug or Alcohol Detox

Cleansing our anatomies appears to be extremely popular. Recently, from diet cleanses to juice cleanses, people are learning how important it is to clear harmful, everyday harmful toxins from our anatomies. Pollutants land within our systems from the meals we eat, what we should drink, and the conditions we reside in.

For anyone who has been slowly taking in or using drugs, they'll likely have higher levels of harmful toxins in their bodies. This may make the detoxing process a fairly dreadful experience if not handled properly.

Just like cleansing your body is resulting in the average individual, it could be even more beneficial for a person who is detoxing from drugs or alcohol.

"Food is an essential medication in restoring health. The earlier a newly-sober person seems great, I've found, the earlier she or he will begin to simply accept a life free from crippling accessories to chemicals - the life span they truly are designed to live." - *Maura Henninger N.D., Huffington*

Post

Nourishment can play a significant role on the path to recovery, as it could help increase the healing procedures inside your body as well as support or lessen the consequences of withdrawal throughout a medication or alcohol detoxification. Let's check out some of the meals and nutritional vitamins that are crucial during a medication or alcohol cleansing:

- **Nutritional vitamins & Minerals**

According to articles published by ***LiveStrong***, *"Zero nutrients, including calcium, iron, magnesium, and zinc, may appear from consuming too many alcoholic beverages for an extended period of your time."* So, it's essential to replenish your body by firmly taking vitamin and nutrient vitamins during detoxification. Getting plenty of the, D, E, K, and B nutritional vitamins, folic acid, calcium, magnesium, and iron are vital vitamins as your body recovers from being malnourished.

- **Fruits & Vegetables**

A lot of people don't consider fruits & vegetables as resources of organic carbs. However, they are excellent sources of dietary fibre to fuel our anatomies with. Dietary fibre has been recognised to help reduce alcoholic beverage's cravings. Not just that, but people who are coping with drug abuse often crave sugars. The fruit is a wholesome way to curb these desires.

- **Protein**

Protein aids your body in repairing cells, as its maintenance is at a cellular level while trying to restore a few of our essential organs. This is important throughout the initial phases of recovery because long term drug abuse can seriously harm organs. Organs like the liver organ, kidneys, heart, and brain all need to go into repair mode on detoxing. Protein also plays a substantial role in blood sugar stabilization, which can help fight cravings. Good causes of protein are available in eggs, chicken, fish, and nuts.

- **Water**

No matter what you might be detoxing from, combating dehydration will be an essential area of the process. Make sure to drink eight 8 cups of water each day. This will not only assist in keeping your body hydrated but also assists in flushing toxins from one's body.

- **Complex Carbohydrates**

Whole grains are a great source of organic carbohydrates, which may be an essential food for detoxing because these types of foods provide energy for your body. The very best complex carbohydrates are available in brown or wild rice, oats, beans, and lentils. These fibre-rich foods move more slowly through the digestive tract, making them a reliable way to obtain energy.

- **Healthy Fats**

These fat and oils provide essential absorption of the nutrients and vitamins the body needs. They are essential for delivering fats into the body, which can result in depressive disorder when deficiencies can be found. Resources of healthy fatty acids include *avocado, coconut oil, flaxseed, nuts, seeds, and essential olive oil.*

- **Super Foods**

Natural foods such as *algae* can play an enormous role in assisting to rid your body of toxins as well as provide energy. The most frequent types of algae are *spirulina* and *chlorella*. Relating to **Dr Mercolla**, *"Chlorella switches into your intestine and binds to the harmful toxins that are released if you are detoxing. It'll bind irreversibly to the toxins and become safely excreted when you have your bowel motion."*

Foods To Avoid During Detox

- **Sugars**

Extreme sugar consumption causes prolonged cravings, lethargy, anxiety, and chemical substance imbalances. In addition, it often creates a fresh kind of addiction for individuals in recovery.

- **Caffeine**

It overstimulates the central nervous system, which can result in panic and insomnia, both of which may be detrimental to a resulting detox and recovery.

Prepared or processed foods such as junk food make the

work of the liver to break down these kinds of food harder because of the preservatives and chemicals within these kinds of foods, hence allow the liver to rest whenever you can during cleansing and early recovery.

Chapter 6
Best Fruits Smoothies for Melting Belly Fat

Sip the right path to slim with these 15 yummy sips. Drink them in the morning, and you will have significantly more energy throughout the day, and eat much less at lunch!

- *Matcha tea natural powder* is the super-slimming key component in this berry drink. Just one single teaspoon helps the body burn belly fat and reduces extra fat cells from forming.

- *The aloe vera juice* in this peachy drink traps toxins and ferries them out of the body, reducing belly bloat. Also, it revs up your metabolism and energy.

- *Blend berries, bananas, and two teaspoons of main maca powder* to improve fat burn off by 18%. You'll lower bad cholesterol by 74%.

- *Probiotic-rich kefir* in this super-powerful OJ smoothie puts the kibosh on fat-promoting inflammation and lowers your threat of weight gain.

Also, it helps to keep you feeling fuller all night.

- Appears like a *frappe* but it's instead a *body fat blaster*. The coconut milk in this formula stimulates the thyroid to make a fat-burning hormone. Your nice tooth and tummy will thank you.

- Besides, its anti-ageing properties, adding *collagen* to your preferred smoothie, can rev up your metabolism and reduce the food cravings hormone.

The result: You'll eat much less and appear great.

- *This tropical-fruit smoothie* can prevent blood-sugar spikes, banish bloat, and help the liver and pancreas concentrate on fat-burning and detoxifying. The simple recipe demands mango, pineapple, and cream of coconut.

- Switch on your brown fat watching calories melt off, because of the hemp proteins in this *kiwi-avocado smoothie* that's as effortless to make as it is to sip.

- We love any banana-berry combo, however, when you add *pea protein*, you lose weight and boost muscle. Another benefit is that the protein lowers your hunger hormone, ghrelin.

- Put in a tablespoon of *chia seed* products to the orange-banana smoothie and change fat-storing cells into fat-burning ones.

  The result: gradual reduction of belly fat.

- Taking *milk* will help you lose two-thirds of the body fat, so you may include yogurt and milk in the raspberry refresher.

- Faster reduction of fat, increased energy, and a brighter feeling after taking in this smoothie each day? Yes, because of *oatmeal*! Observe how to include it in a fruit smoothie here.

- While *proteins* are the fat-burning component in this vanilla-berry smoothie. It's extremely filling up too, so you'll eat much less food at the next meal.

- Blast during that menopot by mixing a tablespoon of *flaxseed* along with *strawberries, kiwi, and yoghurt*. The seed products contain lignans, which tame hot flashes and also have slimming powers.

- Combine one *plum* with a cup of *frozen cherries and Greek yoghurt*, then put in a tablespoon of *chia seeds*. You can get a fat-burning sip that can rev your metabolism and curb food cravings.

Refreshing Raspberry Cream Smoothie

This smoothie packs a nutritional punch filled with antioxidants, healthy fats, magnesium, and probiotics. It's a great snack for between meals or an instant breakfast.

This recipe uses coconut milk yoghurt for the bottom, which is ideal for individuals who are sensitive to milk or have digestive issues; nevertheless, you can also substitute any yogurt of your decision.

Serves 1

Prep time: five minutes

Ingredients

1 cup organic raspberries, iced 6 ounces vanilla-flavoured coconut-milk, yogurt with probiotics, 1 teaspoon Raspberry-Lemon Flavor, 1 cup ice

Directions

Blend all elements until even. Enjoy immediately.

Chapter 7
Breakfast Smoothies for Flat Belly

Recently, I've been on an enormous smoothie kick. I've been making them each morning, and I love the results. The only problem is the time to get ready these 10 flat-belly breakfast smoothies. They're easy to make don't misunderstand me, but I tend to go to snooze several times way too many. Since we have carefully chosen the ingredients to banish belly fat, I don't want to skip the steps.

With a ready-to-blend, the pre-portioned cup filled up with the smoothie ingredients. All you need to do is pop them in the refrigerator until you're prepared to mix away. Then, you just add liquid, and you have a grab-and-go smoothie. I thought this is an excellent idea.

So, making these breakfast smoothies into breakfast packages! It's the perfect, fast and simple way to banish belly fat and start your entire day off right. Each smoothie includes metabolism-boosting substances like *green tea extract, chia seed products, cayenne pepper, flaxseed products, and ginger main.* Add the sweet and creamy tastes of *Greek yoghurt, almond milk, fruits, and vegetables,* and you have a recipe for success!

Feel absolve to make every of these in advance as I did so. It will increase your morning regular routine while still waging battle on belly fat. There's a lot of variety in this set of 10 smooth belly breakfast smoothies that you may make one every day of the week rather than get sick and tired of them!

1. Skinnylicious Proteins Smoothie

Using a protein-packed breakfast is essential if you would like to complete the morning with enough energy to be productive and prevent food craving. This *Skinnylicious Protein Smoothie* is filled with all the nice stuff imaginable: *avocado, baby spinach, Kale, and green tea extract.*

Green tea extract is a casino game changer for banishing belly fat because of its chemical substances called **catechins** that rev in the metabolism.

If you're worried about everything vegetable, don't be! The *spinach and Kale* merge deliciously with the creamy *avocado* and boatload of sweetness from the *apples* and *bananas*.

Ingredients List:

- Avocado.
- Apple.
- Banana.
- Spinach.
- Kale.
- Green Tea

2. Wake Me Up, Keep Me Heading Smoothie

As though the name doesn't say enough, this smoothie is intended to benefit you up even on the slowest moving of mornings. Didn't get enough rest the nighttime before? You may find that, when you certainly feel more energized as you go out the door, you retain that momentum heading the whole day. You can thank the green tea extract for that!

Combined with a variety of fruits and vegetables, along with chia seed products, you'll get a wholesome dose of protein and fibre from energizing superfoods that can keep you awaken and GLOW.

Chia seed products are an excellent option for your top 10 flat belly breakfast smoothies because they contain *omega-3 essential fatty acids* which help lower inflammation.

Ingredients List:

- Banana.
- Grapes.
- Avocado.
- Spinach.
- Kale.
- Chia Seeds.
- Green Tea

3. Kale and Orange Smoothie

This is among the best top 10 flat belly breakfast smoothies if you're looking for something that's bursting with *vitamin C*, which is ideal for maintaining healthy blood sugar.

Orange shines in this smoothie, and pairs incredibly with several juicy fruits and delicious vegetables. The drizzle of honey adds a vitamin dose of sweetness without subjecting your body to artificial sweeteners and processed sugar.

While this smoothie may flavor light, it'll keep you full all night, and that means you can sustain your focus and feel great realizing that you chose an energizing breakfast that's so good for you. The addition of almond milk adds even more fibre and energy-boosting power. At only 131 calories per portion, you can enjoy this creamy, sweet smoothie guilt-free.

Ingredients List:

- Banana.
- Kale.
- Orange.
- Honey.
- Almond Milk

4. Spiced Green Tea Extract Smoothie

Green tea has recently shown up several times in these top 10 flat tummy breakfast smoothies, and with justification. It's a metabolism-boosting agent that health experts tout as a weight-loss miracle.

This smoothie is unlike others in the sense it has quite the kick because of the *cayenne pepper*, which improves the metabolic process to fight belly fat, and combines sensationally with *cinnamon, honey, fruit, and Greek yoghurt*. The result is a creamy, energizing smoothie that will get rid of fat away all early morning long!

Ingredients List:

- Green Tea.
- Cayenne Pepper.
- Ground Cinnamon.
- Honey.
- Pear.
- Apple.
- Orange.

- Greek Yogurt

5. Chocolate Meal Alternative Shake

If sweets for breakfast is your jam, just like a sugary muffin, try out this Chocolate Meal Substitute Tremble instead. It includes a delicate balance of complicated carbs, dietary fibre, and proteins which means you can feel satisfied from the flavor to the consistency to just how it fills you up all early morning long. It's a great introduction for the more magnificent sceptical couple of swapping out breakfast for a dense smoothie since they have this approachable flavor.

Ingredients List:

- Unsweetened Almond Milk.
- Banana.
- Chocolate Proteins Powder.
- Flax Seed

6. Skinny Banana Break up Protein Smoothie

Can a banana break-up smoothie be one of the very best 10 flat-belly breakfast smoothies? It sure can when it's filled with proteins, fruits, and milk product alternatives that combine to produce something that likes indulgent but is so healthy.

This dessert-like smoothie features simple ingredients like *strawberries,* which fight belly fat because they're filled with *polyphenols*, powerful natural chemicals that can stop fat from forming.

Ingredients List:

- Non-fat Greek Yogurt.
- Unsweetened Almond Milk.
- Strawberries.
- Banana.
- Protein Powder

7. Much better than a Tremble - Green Smoothie

This green desire is a mixture of some ingredients we've already covered, like *Banana, Grapes, Kale, and avocado*. It's the addition of ginger that provides it with a kick. *Ginger* is a superb addition to your early morning smoothie, as it is a well-revered fats burner, especially around the belly for a flatter tummy.

The *avocado* adds that smooth, creamy texture which makes for a beautiful drink.

<u>Ingredients List</u>:

- Banana
- Red Grapes.
- Kale.
- Avocado.
- Ginger Root

<u>8. Avocado Pear Smoothie</u>

That is one yummy smoothie that combines sweet and creamy with the fun mixture of *avocado, pear, Greek yoghurt, and raw honey*. Smoothies don't need to have a lot of elements to make sure they are extremely delicious and healthy. Sometimes less is more!

Avocado makes this set of the very best 10 flat tummy breakfast smoothies quite a little because it's rich with healthy fat that is crucial for weight loss.

Ingredients List:

- Greek Yogurt.
- Avocado.
- Raw Honey.
- Vanilla Extract

9. Crazy Blueberry, Mint, and Flax Seed Smoothie

This clean and straightforward smoothie has quite a mixture of belly fat-fighting ingredients. The *blueberries* are rich in *resveratrol*, which is nutritional, and it has beneficial results on the epigenetic systems that trigger putting on weight and fatty liver organs.

Mint is another belly fat fighter, as it could help to keep bloating away.

Ingredients List:

- Flax Seeds.
- Almond Milk.
- Blueberries.
- Honey.

- Mint

10. Superfood Strawberry & Goji Berry Smoothie

Rounding out the set of the very best 10 flat-belly breakfast smoothies is this one fun showcasing *strawberries, honey, and goji berries*.

It's ideal for a person who just can't get along with *spinach and Kale*, which makes it to their morning routine.

Goji berries are great for weight loss because they are rich in several nutritional vitamins that help convert food into energy rather than storing it as body fat.

Ingredients List:

- Goji Berries.
- Strawberries.
- Honey.
- Almond Milk.

If you're seeking to lose weight, especially around your waistline, make healthy decisions from the morning to create the shade for the others of your entire day. These delicious smoothies are a fantastic choice.

Chapter 8
Smoothies For Healthy Digestion

Digestive system isn't the coolest subject, but it's favorite; because a poor Digestive system is the major of so many medical issues and smoothies are one of our go-to breakfasts (*because produce in the morning means organic burgundy or merlot wine later*). Smoothies can be simpler to break down because they're combined (*a few of the work is performed for you*!), but here are some tips to make sure they are even more digestion-friendly.

Steps to make Smoothies Better to Digest

1. ***Chewing:*** makes the human brain resulting in an adequate creation of saliva. Saliva is a complicated combination of electrolytes, bodily hormones, and enzymes essential to break down food. When you have trouble nibbling a smoothie (*it's a strange concept, we obtain it*) transform it into a smoothie dish and perhaps then add toppings like *granola, seed products, nut products, and coconut flakes.*

2. ***Use Steamed Frozen Cauliflower***: Rather than ice, which may be chilling for the digestive tract, use steamed iced cauliflower instead (just put in a little more water if needed). The smoothie won't be quite as chilly.

3. ***Be Careful***: Be familiar with food sensitivities. Keep it non-milk if needed in support of used foods you understand your body enjoys.

4. ***Relax***: Smoothies tend to be considered a grab-and-go kind of food. Do the best you can to relax as you drink (*or eat*!) them, because Digestive system starts in the mind; you should be in a parasympathetic, calm condition to properly process food.

Healthy Digestive System Smoothies

Well-known digestion-friendly smoothie quality recipes boosted with natural probiotics, enzymes, and fibre.

- Mango & Turmeric Healthy Digestive System Smoothie.

- Blueberry & Beet Healthy Digestive system Smoothie.

- Pineapple & Kale Healthy Digestive system Smoothie.

Mango & Turmeric Healthy Digestive system Smoothie

Why It Helps Healthy Digestion

- *Yoghurt or Kefir*: Yogurt and kefir contain probiotics, aka "good" bacteria, to keep your gut healthy. If you're milk-free, opt for unsweetened coconut yoghurt, like GT's Cocoyo.

- *Hemp Seed Products:* Hemp seed products are saturated in both soluble and insoluble dietary fibre, both important to keep the gastrointestinal system regular. Dietary fibre also feeds the probiotics, creating more beneficial bacterias.

- *Turmeric*: Turmeric is a robust anti-inflammatory spice because of the *polyphenol* curcumin. *Curcumin* has been proven to provide therapeutic leads to small studies of inflammatory intestinal disorders.

Ingredients

- 1/2 cup unsweetened milk-free milk.
- 1/2 cup ice.
- 1/2 cup unsweetened yoghurt or kefir (milk-free if desired).
- 1 orange, peel, and white pith removed.
- 1 large carrot, coarsely chopped.
- 1/2 cup iced mango chunks.
- 2 tablespoons of natural hemp seeds.
- 1/4 teaspoon floor turmeric.
- tiny pinch of dark pepper (escalates the bioavailability of the turmeric!).
- pinch of sea salt.

Instructions

- Add all ingredients to a high-speed blender and mix until clean and creamy. Add a little more milk-free milk, if needed, to attain desired consistency.

Blueberry & Beet Healthy Digestive System Smoothie

Why it works with healthy digestion;

- ***Banana***: Bananas contain dietary fibre and prebiotics, which provide gas for the beneficial bacterias in the gut.

- ***Beets***: Beets contain high degrees of folate and manganese, which helps gallbladder function. The gallbladder stores bile, which is vital for the Digestive system and absorption of fat and fat-soluble nutritional vitamins.

- ***Lime Juice***: Like lemons, the acidity of lime juice can help stimulate gastric acid (***HCl***) creation, which is essential to properly break down foods.

- ***Flaxseed***: Flaxseed contains high degrees of gel-forming dietary fibre that goes through the digestive tract without having to be digested, assisting colon detoxification. Just two tablespoons of flaxseed provide about 25% of your daily dietary fibre needs.

Ingredients

- 3/4 cup unsweetened milk-free milk.
- 1/2 cup ice.
- 3/4 cup frozen blueberries.
- 1/2 frozen banana.
- 1 small beet, grated or cut into chunks
- 2 tablespoons of freshly squeezed lime juice.
- 2 tablespoons surface flaxseed.
- 1 pitted Medjool day, optional.
- pinch of sea salt.

Instructions

- Add all ingredients to a high-speed blender and mix until even and creamy. Add a little more milk-free milk, if needed, to attain desired consistency.

Pineapple & Kale Healthy Digestive system Smoothie

Why It Help Healthy Digestion

- ***Pineapple***: Pineapple contains bromelain, a proteolytic and anti-inflammatory enzyme that helps break down foods naturally.

- ***Lemon***: The acidity of lemon juice can help stimulate gastric acid (***HCl***) creation, which is essential to properly break down foods.

- ***Ginger***: Ginger stimulates Digestive system, relieves intestinal gas, relaxes and soothes the digestive tract, and inhibits the forming of inflammatory compounds.

- ***Chia***: Chia seed products are very saturated in dietary fibre, which promotes regularity. Chia seed products also absorb waterand increase in the belly, assisting to keep your senses fuller much longer (*source*).

Ingredients

- 3/4 cup unsweetened milk-free milk.
- 1/2 cup ice.
- 1/2 cup iced pineapple chunks.
- 1/2 frozen banana.
- 1/2 cup coarsely cut Kale.
- 2 tablespoons of freshly squeezed lemon juice.
- 1 teaspoon grated fresh ginger root.
- 2 tablespoons chia seeds.
- 1 pitted Medjool time, optional.
- pinch of sea salt.

Instructions

- Add all ingredients to a high-speed blender and mix until steady and creamy. Add a little more milk-free milk, if needed, to attain desired consistency.

Chapter 9
Green Smoothies That Heal The Gut & Increase Energy

There are benefits to starting your entire day with detoxifying green drinks. Some include clearer pores and skin, deeper rest, less stress, increased energy, a better Digestive system, and improved blood circulation. It is because you're placing cleaning greens into the body that are easy on the digestive tract. The simpler your meal is to break down, the greater energy the body may use towards getting toxins and bacteria out of the body since it isn't using that energy for the Digestive system. That means the body will have time for you to fight the reason for your blemished skin, and the harmful toxins causing it will be flushed out. These detoxifying green beverages are so delicious that you'll undoubtedly enjoy doing all your body a favor!

Belly Cleanser Green Smoothie

Out of the many detoxifying green beverages, I'm going to show you, this is the strongest smoothie. If you aren't used to detoxification drinks whatsoever, I probably wouldn't focus on that one. *Mint is a robust bloodstream detoxifier and reduces bloating.* Lemon detoxes the bloodstream as well, but it additionally flushes harmful toxins from the liver organ, and kidneys and supports digestion. The flavor of relaxing mint pairs perfectly with the lemon in this smoothie, developing a light and delicious green-colored drink.

Ingredients:

- 3 cups water.
- Juice of just one 1 lemon.
- 1 inch little bit of ginger.
- 4 inch little bit of cucumber.
- ¼ cup mint.
- 1-2 handfuls ice.

Directions: Combine all the elements in a blender and mix until smooth.

Cheery Cherry Detoxification Smoothie

This green drink appears red because of the cherries but

contains Kale. Kale is a dark leafy green, and it is very detoxifying to your body. It includes sulfur for liver organ detox, vitamin C for hydrating and replenishing, and dietary fibre for detoxifying your digestive tract. There is undoubtedly lemon juice in this smoothie like the last one, but that one also offers the anti-inflammatory advantages of cherries. *Cherries contain cancer-fighting antioxidants to help you remain healthy.* Chia seed products are also significant detoxifiers, binding to extra water and flushing harmful toxins that are in them.

Ingredients:

- 1 cup iced cherries.
- 2-4 kale cubes or a small number of fresh Kale.
- 1 cup nonmilk milk.
- 2 cups water.
- 2 tablespoons of fresh lemon juice.
- 2 tablespoons chia seed products.
- 1 teaspoon gluten-free vanilla extract

Directions: Combine every one of the substances in a blender and mix until smooth.

Pineapple Ginger Green Detox Smoothie

The frozen pineapple in this green smoothie helps it tastes icy and delicious. It creates the perfect summertime detox breakfast if you ask me. It's not only delicious, but it additionally detoxes the body, improves the digestive system, is anti-inflammatory, and raises circulation. The baby spinach increases immunity, is filled with antioxidants, nutritional vitamins, live enzymes, and is also anti-inflammatory. Fresh ginger provides this smoothie zing with the added advantages of reduced inflammation, improving metabolism and immunity, and bloodstream cleansing.

Ingredients:

- 3 mugs frozen diced pineapple.
- 3 mugs fresh baby spinach.
- 1 cup iced diced banana.
- 1 celery rib (optionally available).
- 1 Grated of fresh ginger (focus on less and add more if desired).
- 1 Tbsp. chia seed products.

Directions: Combine all the elements in a blender and mix until smooth.

Orange Cleansing Drink

I love the flavor of orange in smoothies. You should have no proven fact that you are taking in a healthy cleansing drink if you are eating this thing. What's better still is that you won't have the ability to inform it is green because of the solitary (*yet powerful*!) green leaf added. I've already mentioned the advantages of *fresh ginger, mint, chia seed products, and Kale*. Did you know oranges likewise have detoxifying benefits? It's true; they contain strong antioxidants (*vitamin c*) to help flush harmful toxins and increase your immunity. Oranges are also rich in dietary fibre to help better your Digestive system.

Ingredients:

- 1/2 Banana
- 1 Orange - Peeled
- 1 inch Fresh Ginger
- 1/2 Lime
- 1 Radish

- 1 Tbs Chia Seed products
- 1 Green leaf (Cabbage, Kale, bok choy, Beet leaf)

(Handful Mint Leaves and Stevia to sweeten - Optional)

- 1/2 to at least one 1 Glass of Spring Water- pretty much depending on how thick you prefer it

Directions: Combine every one of the substances in a blender and mix until smooth.

Strawberry Detoxification Green Monster Smoothie

The frozen strawberries get this to an awesome and fresh summer breakfast. However, they contain some amazing detoxifying compounds that produce this green smoothie extra healthy. Strawberries are filled with vitamin C, which can only help you detoxify and clear your skin layer. Vitamin C has been proven to be anti-aging too! So not only will this drink clear your skin layer, but it will help protect it for later. Cucumbers also flush harmful toxins from the body and clear your skin layer.

Ingredients:

- 3/4 cup frozen strawberries

- 1/2 cup cucumber, peeled and sliced up

- One large frozen Banana, damaged into pieces

- 1/2 glass vanilla almond milk (*or alternative milk*)

- 1/2 cups kale, loosely packed, stems removed (*you can also use spinach*)

- Large quantity of spinach

Directions: Combine all the elements in a blender and mix until smooth.

Cleansing Blueberry Monster Smoothie

Don't allow the short substances list or nongreen color of the smoothie to fool you. It is a nutrient-dense powerhouse! I've already talked about how beneficial baby spinach is, but mango and blueberries are fantastic as well. Mango consists of many live digestive enzymes, detoxifying vitamin c, and antioxidants. A mango includes so many enzymes that if you leave pieces on that person and clean it off with tepid to warm water, it can help prevent acne! Blueberries contain an enormous amount of cancer-fighting antioxidants that assist with anti-aging and pores and skin.

Ingredients:

- 1 banana.
- 1/2 cup iced blueberries.
- 1/4 cup frozen mango.
- 1/2 cup excess fat-free Lactaid (*or almond milk*).

Directions: Combine every one of the elements in a blender and mix until smooth.

Basic Kale Detoxification Juice

Although the first smoothie was a robust detoxifier, green juice will defeat away from a smoothie anytime. That's because the nutrition is so condensed and also you don't have any dietary fibre, so it's easy to process. Like I stated before if it's easy to break down, your body may then use its energy to eliminate toxins from the body and clear your skin layer. However, ease of process isn't the only key element. Let's take a look at white grain because it is simple to break down. Yet, this doesn't detoxify the body since it isn't loaded with natural enzymes and nutrition. That's the reason high nutrient content is also important, which green juice definitely will the trick!

Ingredients:

- 5 stalks of Kale or Spinach
- 3 Apples
- 1 Lemon
- 1 Cucumber

Directions: Juice the substances in a juicer. Stress if desired. Makes 16 oz . of juice.

If you add one of the green beverages to your early morning routine, you're sure to see improvements in your skin layer among a great many other things. A significant factor I have noticed is that I do not advocate drinking fluids for several days and I don't think detoxing is wonderful for weight loss. It is just a brief fix, not a lifestyle change, and detoxing should be about eliminating toxins that have developed within you. Cleansing for health, not weight reduction! Perhaps you have ever done detoxification before.

Chapter 9
Smoothies for Radiant Skin

1. The Clear Skin Smoothie

This healthy smoothie recipe, created by Koff, runs on the protein powder produced from hemp seeds, which is a balanced way to obtain skin-boosting *omega-3* and *omega-6* essential fatty acids. The *dandelion greens* are excellent for the liver organ, helping to cleanse your body and skin; the avocado and raw cacao natural powder include a powerful mixture of antioxidants, that help clear the tone and get pores and skin glowing; and the coconut water is packed with potassium, which helps skin cells get the water they have to stay (*and appear*) hydrated.

Blend

- 1 scoop of hemp proteins (Koff likes Manitoba Harvest Hemp Pro 70)
- 1/2 cup organic blueberries
- 1/2 number dandelion greens (*no stems*)
- 11 ounces of coconut water

- 1/4 avocado

- 1 tablespoon uncooked cacao powder.

2. **Banana Almond Flax Smoothie**

This healthy smoothie from Kelly Boyer, owner and Executive Chef of Paleta.com, is filled with skin-loving *plant-based protein, potassium, calcium, dietary fiber, and omega-3s*. The fundamental essential fatty acids in the flaxseed essential oil have anti-inflammatory benefits, which are particularly ideal for red, inflamed, and puffy pores and skin.

Blend

- 1 tablespoon flaxseed essential oil

- 2 tablespoons organic almond butter

- 1 small banana

- 1/2 cup organic apple juice

- 1 cup of ice cubes

3. **Mango Yogurt Smoothie**

Boyer also created this healthy smoothie and said the frozen mango offers its sweetness and clean texture and gives skin-boosting nutritional vitamins B6, C and E. Plus, the omega-3s in the seafood oil help regulate oil creation, which increases hydration, aids in preventing acne, and staves off lines and wrinkles.

Blend

- 1 tbsp fish essential oil
- 1/2 cup simple, low-fat, organic yogurt
- 1/2 cup iced mango chunks
- 1/2 cup orange juice
- 1/2 cup ice.
- 1 fresh mint leaf (*optionally available*)

4. **Very Berry Detoxification Smoothie**

The powerful mixture of antioxidants in this healthy smoothie (also created by Boyer) helps cleanse your liver, which processes the toxins that may be contributing to your skin layer woes. Reward: It's a terrific way to sneak in a few bitter-tasting greens because the berry taste overpowers the flavor of the vegetables.

Blend

- 1 tablespoon fish essential oil
- 1/4 cup frozen strawberries
- 1/4 cup frozen blueberries
- 1/4 cup frozen raspberries
- 1/4 cup frozen banana
- 1/4 cup chopped kale leaves
- 1 cup of filtered water

5. **Coconut-Pear Dream Smoothie**

Hemp milk is a superb alternative to milk products, as milk products can contribute to skin irritation in a few people. This easy, delicious smoothie recipe was made by Manitoba Harvest, a hemp foods company. Nevertheless, you may use any non-milk alternative.

Blend

- 1/2 cup hemp milk
- 1/2 cup coconut milk or coconut water
- one to 2 tablespoons vanilla proteins natural powder (preferably Manitoba Harvest Organic Vanilla)
- 1 pear, peeled and cored
- Couple of spinach or Kale
- A splash of coconut extract (*to get more coconut taste*).
- 1 cup ice

6. **Berry Blast**

Academy of Nourishment and Dietetics spokesperson *Angela Ginn* created this healthy smoothie, which seeks to protect your skin layer from harmful contaminants by using antioxidants. "The omega 3 essential fatty acids (*within the flaxseed*) put in a protecting layer to your skin to keep the toxins and bacteria out,". "Beautiful pores and skin start from the within."

Blend

- 1 cup almond milk

- 2 scoops of hemp powder
- 1 cup frozen combined berries
- 1/2 fresh spinach
- 1 tablespoon of grounded flaxseed
- 1/2 banana
- Add ice as desired

7. **Strawberry-Banana Smoothie**

This healthy smoothie is focused on fighting the signals of aging. The strawberries within the anti-aging elixir contain vitamin C, an all-natural collagen contractor. "Collagen is the structural element of the skin we have and helps maintain our skin easy and supple,". "Vitamin C also functions as an antioxidant that protects against and helps repair the skin we have from harm done by super violet light and free radicals."

Blend

- 4 ounces Greek yoghurt
- 1/4 cup milk (or milk alternative)
- 1 tablespoon floor flax seed

- 1/2 cup iced strawberries, about 5-6
- 1/2 medium, ripe Banana

8. Tropical Fruits Smoothie with Coconut Water

If you'd like glowing skin (*and a tropical getaway in a glass*), this healthy smoothie is perfect for you. Relating to Haas, dehydration is a significant player in pores and skin dullness, and the trick to flawless pores and skin is keeping it nice and hydrated. "This smoothie hydrates in two ways,". "First, with the coconut drinking water, and then with all that water that's normally within the fruits. Hydration never tasted so excellent!" You have that right.

Blend

- 4 ounces Greek yoghurt
- 1/4 cup coconut water
- 1/2 cup iced, diced mango
- 1/2 cup freezing, diced pineapple
- 1/2 medium, ripe Banana
- Optionally available add-in: 1/4 cup loaded shredded carrot

9. **Chocolate-Cherry Smoothie**

Who doesn't love a wholesome smoothie which involves chocolates? Another concoction created by Haas, this smoothie battles fine lines and increases your skin's shine.

The flavonoids at night chocolates are natural antioxidants that create skin smoother and softer and help protect you against sunburn and UV harm. "In addition they increase blood circulation to your skin, providing an all-natural, rosy shine,". "Make sure to look for at least 70% cacao to get the most pores and skin benefits, though." You may never feel bad about eating delicious chocolate again. You're pleasant.

Blend

- 4 ounces Greek yogurt
- 1 tablespoon cocoa powder
- 1/4 cup milk (or milk alternative)
- 1/2 cup iced, sweet cherries
- 1/2 medium, ripe Banana
- 1/2 cup packed spinach

10. Green Tea Extract Cooler

Created by **Mary Kennedy**, M.S., nourishment and wellbeing professional who works for Stonyfield Plantation, this healthy smoothie combines two powerful skin foods: organic yoghurt and green tea extract. The yogurt is packed with live energetic cultures offering the gut with beneficial bacterias, which helps Digestive system (*the better your digestive system operates, the better your skin layer can look*); mint and honey also help fight "bad" bacterias, and the green tea extract is packed with anti-aging antioxidants.

Blend

- 1 cup Stonyfield organic fat-free key lime yoghurt
- 1 cup prepared green tea extract, cooled
- 1/2 cup loosely packed mint, chopped
- Juice and zest of 2 limes
- 1 teaspoon honey
- 2 cups ice

11. Sour Apple Smoothie

This smoothie, also created by Kennedy, uses flaxseed oil, which is rich with omega-3 essential fatty acids that are advantageous for skin health.

Blend

- 1 Granny Smith apple, cored and chopped
- 1 banana
- 1 cup of orange juice
- 1 cup Oikos Organic Vanilla Greek Yogurt
- 1/2 cup Stonyfield organic fat-free milk
- 1 tablespoon flaxseed essential oil

12. Sweet & Salty Chai Lassi

Billy Brigtsen, a chef in NEW YORK, created this smoothie recipe using skin-healing spices.

Blend

- 3 green cardamom pods, crushed
- 3 black peppercorns
- 3 cloves
- 1 entire allspice berry
- 1/2 tablespoon grated ginger
- 1 cup of water

Directions:

Place the above elements in a little container and simmer for a few moments, until the water is reduced to 1/4 glass. Cool, then mix with:

- 16 ounces Green Valley Organics kefir
- 4 tablespoon maple syrup

13. Fruit Fusion

Antioxidants also assist in preventing blemishes. So if you

would like radiant and clear pores and skin, we recommend attempting this supercharged smoothie. Filled up with anti-aging antioxidants like nutritional vitamins C and E, this healthy smoothie is a diet powerhouse made to leave your skin layer glowing. "The zinc in the smoothie can also help heal rashes, reduce irritation, and prevent blocked skin pores," Ginn says. "The selenium within the flaxseed also may help to reduce the chance of malignancy."

Blend

- 1 cup of coconut milk
- 1/2 cup papaya
- 1/2 cup iced pineapples
- 1/2 banana
- 1/2 Ripe avocado (*peeled*)
- 1 tablespoon of grounded flaxseed
- 2 scoops of hemp powder
- Add glaciers as desired

14. Creamy Orange Creamsicle Smoothie

More hemp plus vitamin C-rich orange and healthy fat-filled avocado makes this healthy smoothie formula a great option to a sugar-filled dessert.

<u>Blend</u>

- 1 cup hemp milk
- 1-2 tablespoons hemp proteins powder -- preferably vanilla-flavored
- 1 orange (peeled and chopped up)
- 1/2 avocado (peeled and sliced up)

15. <u>Noni Colada</u>

Coconut water kefir is another excellent nonmilk smoothie ingredient, and it's packed with probiotics the "good" bacteria that help to keep our digestion running well (*and the skin we have clear because of this*). The pineapple in this smoothie formula, created by organic vegan. **Chef Jason Andrew Wrobel**, also works as an anti-inflammatory agent, assisting to calm puffy, annoyed skin.

<u>Blend</u>

- 10 ounces coconut water kefir.

- Handful of ice.
- 4 ounces frozen pineapple chunks.
- 1 teaspoon dried noni fruits powder.
- 1/8 teaspoon surface cinnamon.
- 1/8 teaspoon floor nutmeg.
- Pinch of sea salt.
- Sweetener to flavor (15% dropper-full of vanilla stevia is fantastic).

Chapter 10

Smoothies For Weight Loss and Body Detox

1. Metabolism Booster Green Cleansing Smoothie

The Thing You Need:

- 1/2 avocado
- 1 kiwi
- 1 celery stick
- 1 tablespoon sunflower seed powder
- A small number of mint leaves
- Newly ground peppercorns
- Salt

How To Prepare

- Scoop the avocado flesh out and cut it into medium-sized cubes.
- Peel off the kiwi, toss it, and combine it with the avocado cubes into the blender.

- Slice the celery stay in two and toss it into the blender.

- Put in a few mint leaves, sunflower seed powder, and a pinch of sodium and present it as a spin.

- Then add freshly surface peppercorn before you drink the smoothie.

Benefits

- Avocados are rich in antioxidants such as neoxanthin, chrysanthemaxanthin, lutein, vitamin E, and vitamin C.

- The phytonutrients and vitamins within kiwi help protect the **DNA** from harm, scavenge harmful free radicals, guard against arthritis, asthma, cancer of the colon, macular degeneration, and improve cardiovascular health.

- Celery is an excellent way to obtain antioxidants that protect you from gastrointestinal swelling, atherosclerosis, and various kinds of cancer.

- Mint is rich in nutritional vitamins A, C, and B-complex, and nutrients such as magnesium, iron, and calcium mineral. It works with the digestive tract and prevents microbial contamination and cell harm.

2. **Fruity Kale Cleansing Smoothie**

The Thing You Need:

- 4 baby kale leaves
- 1/2 cup green grapes
- 1/2 grapefruit
- 1/2 cup watermelon
- A small number of mint leaves
- 1/2 teaspoon pepper
- A pinch of salt

How To Prepare

- Clean all the fruits before you cut or juice them.
- Blend the baby kale leaves, watermelon, grapes, and some mint leaves.
- Add the juice of half of a grapefruit, a pinch of sodium, pepper, and mix well.

Benefits

- Kale is a great source of nutritional vitamins A, C, and K, copper, manganese, calcium mineral, potassium, and soluble fiber. These help lower cholesterol, help weight reduction, improve cardiovascular health insurance, and fight malignancy.

- Grapes are a good way to obtain nutritional vitamins K, B2, and C, and copper. The resveratrol within grapes takes on an essential role in increasing longevity. Grapes also regulate blood sugar, improve cognitive functions, and drive back microbial infections.

- Watermelons contain lycopene that enhances cardiovascular health insurance and cucurbitacin E that scavenges reactive o2 radicals. The part nearest to the rind gets the finest focus of antioxidants, vitamin C, and flavonoids. This helps reduces weight, relax the muscles, and control blood circulation pressure.

- Grapefruit scavenges free air radicals, thus assisting in battle malignancy and lower bloodstream cholesterol. Also, it aids weight reduction.

- Mint helps the digestive tract, prevents microbial illness, and prevents cellular damage.

3. **Spinach Cucumber Chilling Detox Smoothie**

The Thing You Need:

- 1 cup spinach leaves
- 1/2 cucumber
- 1/2 lemon
- A small number of mint leaves
- 1/2 teaspoon roasted cumin powder
- Salt

How To Prepare

- Take away the stems, roughly chop the spinach leaves and cucumber and toss them in a blender.
- Toss in a small number of mint leaves and put in a pinch of sodium. Give it a spin.
- To help make the roasted cumin natural powder, take two tablespoons of cumin seed products and fry them without essential oil in a frying skillet. Grind the roasted cumin seed products and store them

within an airtight cup jar.

- Transfer the spinach smoothie to a cup, add the juice of half of a lemon and half of a teaspoon of roasted cumin natural powder. Stir well.

Benefits

- Spinach is a great source of nourishment. It protects you from numerous kinds of malignancy, mascular degeneration, and strengthens bone fragments.

- Cucumbers are rich in lignans such as pinoresinol, *lariciresinol,* and *secoisolariciresinol* which improve cardiovascular health. The cucurbitacins A, B, C, D, and E help to combat cancer.

- Mint is rich in vitamin A, vitamin C, vitamin B-complex, and nutrients such as magnesium, iron, and calcium mineral. It works with the digestive tract, prevents microbial disease, and prevents cellular damage.

- Lemons are a good way to obtain vitamin C, which protects against arthritis rheumatoid, supports the Digestive system, and fights the mouth area, breast, skin, and cancer of the colon.

- Cumin seed products are rich in iron and assist in the forming of red blood cellular material and aid the Digestive system and weight reduction.

4. **Vegan Cleansing & Fat Burn off Smoothie**

The Thing You Need:

- 1/2 cup baby carrots
- 1 tomato
- 1 celery
- 1/2 lemon juice
- A small number of coriander leaves
- 1 teaspoon roasted cumin seed powder
- Newly ground pepper
- Salt

How To Prepare

- Clean all the vegetables.
- Chop the baby carrots, tomato, celery, and coriander leaves and toss them into a blender and present it a

spin.

- Fry two tablespoons of cumin seed products without essential oil in a frying skillet. Grind the roasted cumin seed products and store them within an airtight cup jar.

- Transfer the smoothie to a cup and add the juice of half of a lemon, just a little freshly floor pepper, and a pinch of sodium. Stir well.

Benefits

- Carrot is rich in nutritional vitamins A, K, C, biotin, dietary fibre, antioxidants, and nutrients. It can help to enhance the heart and eye health insurance and lower the chance of cancer of the colon.

- Tomatoes are rich in lycopene, which boosts bone health. Fresh tomato vegetables lower bloodstream cholesterol and the chance of atherosclerosis and guard against numerous kinds of malignancy.

- Celery is an excellent way to obtain antioxidants that drive back gastrointestinal irritation, atherosclerosis, and various kinds of cancer.

- Lemons are an excellent way to obtain vitamin C

that helps drive back rheumatoid arthritis, aids digestion, and battles mouth, breast, pores and skin, and cancer of the colon.

- Cumin seed products are rich in iron. They help the forming of red bloodstream cells, support the Digestive system and weight reduction, and drive back liver and abdomen cancer.

- Coriander leaves have high vitamin A and vitamin K content. Also, they are rich in nutrients such as calcium mineral and potassium. Coriander leaves are helpful in dealing with indigestion, curing skin and menstrual disorders, keeping blood sugars and cholesterol levels, and enhancing vision.

5. Coconut Water& Berries Cleansing Smoothie

The Thing You Need:

- 1 glass soft coconut water
- 1/2 cup tender coconut
- 1 cup strawberries
- 1 mid-sized gooseberry

- 2 blueberries
- Mint leaves

How To Prepare

- Toss the tender coconut, strawberries, blueberries, and mint leaves into a blender.
- Carefully remove the seed from the gooseberry, cut into four pieces and throw into the blender and present it a spin.
- Add the coconut water into the blender and spin it for three seconds.
- Pour it into a cup and enjoy!

Benefits

- Tender coconut water is a great way to obtain electrolytes, vitamins, protein, and fiber. It can help to regulate blood sugar, aids weight reduction, and cleanses the digestive tract.
- Strawberries are rich in vitamin C, manganese, and dietary fiber. These red and luscious fruits have antioxidant and anti-inflammatory properties. Also, they assist in regulating blood sugar.

- Gooseberries contain vitamins, nutrients, antioxidants, and fibre. These assist in improving skin, curly hair, and heart health insurance and increase immunity.

- Blueberries are rich in antioxidants that assist in improving brain function, cardiovascular health, and vision health, regulate blood sugar and drive back cancer.

- Mint aids the Digestive system and prevents microbial infections.

6. Sweet & Tangy Fruits Smoothie

The Thing You Need:

- 5 lychees
- 1/2 cup pineapple
- 1/2 apple
- 1/2 pomegranate
- 1/2 cup papaya
- 1/2 cup green grapes

- Lemon juice
- 1/2 teaspoon dark salt
- Mint leaves

How To Prepare

- Clean all the fruits before chopping.
- Slice the apple and get rid of the seed products.
- Take the seed products from the lychees.
- Throw in all the fruits and mint leaves into the blender and present it as a spin.
- Put in a dash of lemon juice and black color salt. Mix well.

Benefits

- Pineapple contains cysteine proteases that assist in digesting protein. Also, it contains bromelain, which not only aids the Digestive system but also functions as an anti-inflammatory agent.
- Apples are nutrition-dense fruits that help guard against asthma attacks, battle malignancy, and regulate blood sugar.

- Lychees contain oligonol that prevents viral infections, helps weight reduction, and improves blood flow.

- Pomegranate helps prevent type II diabetes, malignancy (*prostate and breasts*), and cardiovascular disease. Additionally, it is beneficial for individuals who suffer from arthritis, blood circulation pressure, pores and skin diseases, and cognitive disorders. It increases memory and blood flow.

- Papaya is a high source of nutritional vitamins, minerals, & most importantly, papain, the digestive enzyme. It can help to fight constipation, makes the heart more powerful, and also battles cancer of the colon.

- Lemons are a good way to obtain vitamin C that works with Digestive system and helps combat numerous kinds of malignancy.

- Mint aids Digestive system and prevents microbial infections and cellular damage.

7. Banana Passion Cleansing Smoothie

The Thing You Need:

- 1 banana
- 1 passion fruit
- 1 cup milk
- 1 teaspoon flaxseed powder
- 1 teaspoon flaked almond
- A pinch of salt

How To Prepare

- Peel and slice the Banana and toss into the blender.
- Slice the passion fruit and scoop out the fruit into the blender.
- Add the milk, natural flaxseed powder, flaked almonds, and a pinch of sodium and
- give it a spin.

Benefits

- Bananas are rich in potassium that helps to regulate blood circulation pressure. The sterols in bananas help with keeping a check-up on cholesterol levels in the bloodstream. Bananas are also a good way to obtain soluble fibre that helps in the Digestive system as well as weight reduction.

- Flaxseeds have a higher polyphenol antioxidant content, which helps to detoxify your body. They also help weight reduction, prevent cardiovascular diseases, as well as lower insulin levels of resistance.

- Passion fruits are rich in nutritional vitamins A and C, fibre, nutrients, and antioxidants. It can help fight dental and lung malignancies, regulates blood circulation pressure, shield against flu, and helps to maintain good cellular membrane health.

- Milk is a superb source of calcium mineral, protein, body fat, and good carbs. Milk helps to strengthen bone fragments and regulate blood circulation pressure.

- Almonds help lower cholesterol levels and guard against diabetes and high blood circulation pressure.

8. Ginger & Fruits Cleansing Drink

The Thing You Need:

- 1/2 inch ginger root

- 1 orange
- 1 kiwi
- 1 cup of green grapes
- Mint leaves
- A pinch of dark salt

How To Prepare

- Clean the ginger main thoroughly and scrape the peel from the lime utilizing a knife.
- Slice the ginger main and toss it into the blender.
- Peel off the orange and kiwi and toss them into the blender.
- Toss in the green grapes and some mint leaves. Give it a spin.
- Transfer the smoothie to a cup, put in a pinch of black colored salt, and mix well.

Benefits

- Ginger is utilized in many tasty recipes and is an excellent way to obtain antioxidants. They have anti-inflammatory properties and soothes the gastrointestinal tract.

- The phytonutrients and vitamins within kiwi help protect the DNA from harm, scavenge harmful free radicals, guard against arthritis, asthma, cancer of the colon, and macular degeneration, and improve cardiovascular health.

- Grapes are a good way to obtain copper and nutritional vitamins K, B2, and C. They contain resveratrol, which helps boost the lifespan. Grapes also regulate blood sugar, improve cognitive functions, and drive back microbial infections.

- Oranges are filled with vitamin C and dietary fiber. This makes them a great way to obtain antioxidants. Oranges also lower bloodstream cholesterol levels, prevent kidney rock formation, decrease the threat of ulcers, tummy, and lung malignancy, and drive back arthritis rheumatoid, and cardiovascular diseases.

- Mint is rich in vitamin A, vitamin C, vitamin B-complex, and nutrients such as magnesium, iron, and calcium mineral. Mint facilitates the digestive tract and stops microbial infections and cell harm.

9. Garlic clove & Spinach Cleansing Smoothie

The Thing You Need:

- 1 cup spinach
- 2 cloves of garlic
- 1/4 cup boiled nice corn
- 1/2 lime
- A pinch of salt

How To Prepare

- Clean the spinach leaves thoroughly, chop them roughly, and toss them into the blender.
- Peel the garlic clove cloves and toss them into the blender.
- Toss in the boiled nice corn and add the juice of half of a lime.
- Put in a pinch of salt and present it as a spin.

Benefits

- Spinach is an extremely nutritious food. It battles against malignancy, strengthens bone fragments, and prevents macular degeneration.

- Garlic helps to battle malignancy, metabolize iron, and stop microbial infections.

- Nice corns are rich in carotenoids, fibre, and vitamins that help regulate blood sugar and support digestion.

- Lime is very useful in regulating the Digestive system. It can help with gastritis, heartburn, and constipation.

10. Liver Cleansing Smoothie

The Thing You Need:

- 1 grapefruit
- 1 cup baby carrots
- 3 broccoli florets
- 1 celery
- 1 green tea extract bag
- 1 tablespoon honey

- 1 teaspoon roasted cumin powder
- Mint leaves for garnishing
- A pinch of salt

How To Prepare

- Chop the baby carrots, celery, and broccoli florets and throw them into a blender.
- Boil water and drop the green tea extract bag for 5 minutes. Add the green tea herb to the blender.
- Toss in the grapefruit, honey, roasted cumin natural powder, and a pinch of sodium and present it a spin.
- Garnish with mint leaves.

Benefits

- Grapefruit is rich in vitamin C and lycopene (*an anti-cancer agent*). It decreases cholesterol, cleanses the liver organ, has antioxidant properties, and prevents the forming of kidney rocks.
- Carrots assist in weight reduction, improve vision, increase cardiovascular health, and also combat cancer.

- Honey contains an array of minerals and vitamins, and it can help in metabolizing cholesterol and essential fatty acids and supports the Digestive system.

- Green tea increases immunity and is an excellent way to obtain catechins, which are a kind of antioxidant. They scavenge the harmful oxygen radicals, therefore slowing down maturing and avoiding the proliferation of malignancy cells.

- Cumin seed products are rich in iron and assist in the forming of red bloodstream cells. In addition, they aid the Digestive system and weight reduction and drive back liver and belly cancer.

- Celery helps to soothe the digestive system and protects from cancer of the colon and atherosclerosis.

- Broccoli has antioxidant and anti-inflammatory properties, which will make it the best detoxifier. It helps digestion and enhances centre health.

11. Colon Facial cleanser Smoothie

The Thing You Need:

- ½ lemon juice

- 1 apple

- 1 cup spinach

- Pinch of salt

- Pinch of cayenne pepper

How To Prepare

- Chop the apple and spinach and toss into a blender.

- Add the lemon juice and present it as a spin.

- Mix in a pinch of sodium and cayenne pepper before taking in.

Benefits

- Apples are rich in antioxidants, phytochemicals, and soluble fibre. They assist in weight reduction, drive back cardiovascular diseases, and stop uncontrolled cell departments.

- Spinach helps lose weight by increasing satiety, lowering food cravings, and mobilizing body fat.

- Lemons raise the enzymes involved with ßoxidation, therefore it helps to mobilize body fat.

12. Negative Calorie Smoothie

The Thing You Need:

- 2 stalks of celery
- ½ grapefruit
- ½ cup cut Kale
- ½ beetroot
- ½ teaspoon dark salt

How To Prepare

- Chop the celery stalks and beetroot. Toss into the blender.
- Add the grapefruit juice and Kale to the blender and present it a spin.
- Pour it into a cup, add black sodium, and mix well.

Benefits

- Celery is a low-calorie veggie that helps to lose weight by increasing satiety and utilizing stored body fat as energy to handle your body functions.

- *Beetroots* are an affluent source of nutritional vitamins, nutrients, antioxidants, and other phytonutrients that assist in improving immunity and reduce coronary disease risk.
- Eating grapefruit juice helps to reduce weight and also raises insulin sensitivity.
- Kale lowers **LDL** levels in the bloodstream, is a wealthy source of fibre, and prevents cardiovascular diseases.

13. Tangy Stomach Fat Burner

The Thing You Need:

- ¼ lemon
- ½ orange
- 1 carrot
- ½ cup cut leek
- ¼ in. gingerroot
- 1 teaspoon apple cider vinegar

- Pinch of salt

How To Prepare

- Approximately chop the carrot and ginger. Toss into the blender.

- Add chopped leek, orange, and lemon juice. Give it a spin.

- Pour into a cup and add apple cider vinegar and sodium.

- Stir well.

Benefits

- Carrots are rich in antioxidants and phytonutrients that help drive back poor eyesight, atherosclerosis, and malignancy.

- Oranges are a good way to obtain vitamin C that helps increase immunity and lose weight.

- Leeks include a substantial amount of polyphenols that help reduce weight, protect against diabetes, allergic reactions, and arthritis rheumatoid.

- Ginger is rich in antioxidants, nutritional vitamins,

and has anti-inflammatory properties. It helps the Digestive system and works effectively against motion sickness and nausea.

- Lemons are rich in vitamin C and it does increase the degrees of enzymes that assist in body fat metabolism.

14. Fenugreek & Plum Metabolism Stimulator

The Thing You Need:

- 2 teaspoon fenugreek seeds
- 1 plum
- 4-5 mint leaves

How To Prepare

- Soak the fenugreek seed products overnight in a glass of water.
- Each day, strain the water and dispose of the seeds.
- Chop the plum and toss it into a blender.
- Add the mint leaves and fenugreek seed products soaked water.

- Give it a spin.

Benefits

- Fenugreek seed products have lipid decreasing and antioxidant properties. In addition, it prevents lipid and blood sugar absorption.

- Plums have phytonutrients that assist in the absorption of iron, reducing blood glucose and bad cholesterol levels.

- Mint leaves soothe the digestive system, helps in decreasing bad cholesterol and blood circulation pressure, and effectively relieve muscle pain.

15. Stay Energetic Smoothie

The Thing You Need:

- ½ glass red grapes
- ¼ cup banana
- 4 soaked almonds
- ¼ cup raspberry

- Pinch of dark salt

How To Prepare

1. Toss the reg grapes, Banana, raspberries, and almonds into a blender.

2. Give it a spin and put it into a cup.

3. Put in a pinch of dark salt and mix well.

Benefits

- Grapes have antimicrobial, antioxidant, anti-inflammatory, and anticancer properties. Also, it decreases aging and lowers blood sugar.

- Though bananas may appear like fattening food, they have numerous other health advantages that indirectly aid weight loss. It is rich in minerals and vitamins, stimulates the Digestive system, prevents cardiovascular diseases, and boosts muscle power.

- Sweet and sour raspberries are rich in antioxidants and also have anti-inflammatory properties. It is an anti-obesity agent and helps to control blood sugar.

- Almonds are rich in healthy excess fat and also offer a probiotic impact thereby supporting the proper

Digestive system of food.

16. Cucumber And Orange Cleansing Smoothie

The Thing You Need:

- ½ cup cucumber
- 1 orange
- 1 green tea extract bag
- 2 mint leaves

How To Prepare

- Dip the green tea extract bag into half of a glass of warm water. Let it cool off to room heat.
- Toss the cucumber, orange, and teas into a blender and present it as a spin.
- Pour into a cup.
- Garnish with mint leaves.

Benefits

- Green tea helps to guard against diabetes, obesity, and cardiovascular diseases.

- Cucumbers are a low-calorie and high-water content veggie that helps to lower lipid levels and has anti-diabetic results.

- Oranges are a full source of vitamin C, really help to lower blood circulation pressure, protects from asthma, joint disease, and hearing infections.

- Mint leaves have anti-inflammatory and antioxidant properties offering safety against digestive problems relieves muscle pain and helps to soothe your skin.

17. Fruits & Nut Cleansing Smoothie

The Thing You Need:

- 1 cup apple
- 2 dates
- 4 soaked almonds
- ½ glass fat-free milk
- 1 teaspoon of cocoa powder

How To Prepare

1. Approximately chop the apple and times.

2. Toss the apple, schedules, milk, and almonds into a blender and present it as a spin.

3. Pour into a cup and dirt the cocoa natural powder on top.

<u>Benefits</u>

- Apples are rich in flavonoids, carotenoids, phenolics, nutritional vitamins, minerals, and soluble fibre that help to drive back cardiovascular diseases, decrease bad cholesterol and decrease the threat of diabetes and asthma.

- Times are a high source of nutritional vitamins B-complex and C, carotenoids, phenolics, and fibre. They have anti-inflammatory, anticancer, and anti-hemorrhagic properties.

- Almonds are rich in healthy fats, nutrients, and phytonutrients. It can help to reduce the chance of oxidative stress, weight problems, diabetes, and sugar homeostasis.

- Milk is a rich source of calcium minerals and helps to strengthen bone fragments, reduces the chance of cardiovascular diseases, putting on weight, and diabetes.

18. Muscle Activator Cleansing Smoothie

The Thing You Need:

- 1 cup spinach
- 2 tablespoon low-fat yogurt
- ¼ glass mung bean sprouts
- 5 mint leaves
- Pinch of dark salt

How To Prepare

1. Toss the spinach, mung bean sprouts, mint leaves, and low-fat yogurt into the blender and present it a spin.

2. Pour into a cup and put in a pinch of dark salt.

3. Stir well.

Benefits

- Spinach helps to lose weight by increasing satiety,

lowering food cravings, and mobilizing body fat.

- Mung beans are saturated in protein content and for that reason can be viewed as muscle food. Additionally, it is rich in vitamin K, folate, calcium mineral, and phosphorus.

- Yogurt is creamy with good gut bacterias that assist in digestion, calcium mineral, potassium, magnesium, and vitamin B-12.

- Mint leaves have anti-inflammatory and antioxidant properties that battle digestive issues, relieve muscle pain, and help to soothe your skin.

19. Digestion Grasp Blaster

The Thing You Need:

- 1 cup buttermilk
- 1 teaspoon fennel seeds
- 1 teaspoon cumin seeds
- ¼ cup blueberries
- ¼ inches ginger root

- Pinch of dark salt

How To Prepare

- Make use of a mortar and pestle to grind the cumin and fennel seed products.

- Toss the blueberries and ginger into a blender and present it as a spin.

- Pour it into a cup.

- Add buttermilk and surface cumin-fennel seeds. Mix well.

Benefits

- Buttermilk assists with digestion by giving the gut good bacterias. In addition, it has diuretic properties.

- Blueberries are rich in vitamins, nutrients, and soluble fibre. It helps to lessen stomach fat, reduces the chance of Type II diabetes, helps prevent atherosclerosis, and increases memory.

- Cumin seeds help digestion, prevent cardiovascular disease, which is best for your eyesight.

- Fennel seeds, aside from being truly a flavoring agent, assist in the Digestive system, fighting cold, and it is a highly effective menstruation promoter.

- Ginger is rich in antioxidants, nutritional vitamins, and has anti-inflammatory properties. It helps the Digestive system and works effectively against motion sickness and nausea.

20. Rejuvenator Detoxification Smoothie

The Thing You Need:

- ¼ cup tomato
- ½ cup watermelon
- ½ cup sensitive coconut water
- Pinch of dark salt

How To Prepare

- Toss the tomato and watermelon into a blender and present it as a spin.
- Pour into a cup.
- Add coconut waterand a pinch of dark salt.
- Stir well.

Benefits

- Tomato can be an anti-cancer agent, it helps you to drive back cardiovascular diseases, unhealthy weight, high blood circulation pressure, and diabetes.

- Watermelon helps to rehydrate cellular material and keeps unlimited cellular proliferation in balance, prevents cardiovascular diseases, diabetes, and enhances vision.

- Coconut water is rich in natural electrolytes, looked after assists with lipid mobilization.

21. Pomegranate And Guava Detoxification Smoothie

The Thing You Need:

- ½ cup pomegranate
- ½ glass ripe guava
- 1 teaspoon floor flax seeds
- Pinch of salt

How To Prepare

1. Mix the pomegranate and guava utilizing a blender.

2. Pour it into a cup and add surface flax seed and sodium.

3. Stir well.

Benefits

- Pomegranate helps to lower high blood circulation pressure and bad cholesterol levels, has antioxidant, anticancer, and anti-inflammatory properties.

- Guavas are rich in dietary fibre and potassium. It can help to lower bloodstream lipid and high blood circulation pressure.

- Flax seeds help decrease the lipid levels in the bloodstream and also protects against cardiovascular diseases.

22. Passion Fruits And Cucumber Detoxification Smoothie

The Thing You Need:

- 1 passion fruit
- 1 cup cucumber
- Mint leaves
- Pinch of dark salt

How To Prepare

1. Scoop the enthusiastic fruits out and toss them into a blender.

2. Add cucumber and mint leaves to the blender.

3. Give it a spin.

4. Pour into a cup and put in a pinch of dark salt. Mix well.

Benefits

- Passion fruits are rich in minerals, nutritional vitamins, antioxidants, and fibre. It is a laxative and helps to maintain healthy skin and mucous membranes.
- Cucumbers contain nutritional vitamins, nutrients,

and phytonutrients that help soothe pores and skin, lower lipid levels, can be an antidiabetic agent, and stop constipation.

- Mint leaves soothe the digestive system, helps lower bad cholesterol and blood circulation pressure, and provides effectual relief from muscle pain.

23. Pumpkin Seed products And Strawberry Detoxification Smoothie

The Thing You Need:

- 1 cup strawberry
- 2 teaspoon floor pumpkin seed
- Pinch of dark salt

How To Prepare

- Grind the strawberry in a blender.
- Pour into a cup.
- Add surface pumpkin seed and a pinch of dark salt.
- Stir well.

Benefits

- Strawberries are rich in vitamin C, manganese, and dietary fibre. These red and luscious fruits have antioxidant and anti-inflammatory properties. In addition, they assist in regulating blood sugar.

- Pumpkin seeds help regulate insulin levels and offer security against diabetes. It does increase good cholesterol levels and soothes menstrual cramps.

24. Kiwi And Spinach Detoxification Smoothie

The Thing You Need:

- 2 kiwis
- ½ cup spinach
- 1 tablespoon lime juice
- Pinch of salt

How To Prepare

- Peel off and roughly chop the kiwis.
- Toss the kiwi and spinach into a blender.
- Mix well and put into a cup.

- Add lime juice and a pinch of sodium. Stir well.

Benefits

- The phytonutrients and vitamins within kiwi protect the DNA from harm, scavenge harmful free radicals, provide protection from arthritis, asthma, cancer of the colon, macular degeneration, and improve cardiovascular health.

- Spinach is a great source of diet. It protects you from numerous kinds of malignancy, macular degeneration, and strengthens bone fragments.

- The lime helps to regulate the Digestive system. It helps relieve gastritis, heartburn, and constipation.

25. Green Apple And Avocado Detoxification Smoothie

The Thing You Need:

- 1 cup green apple
- ¼ cup avocado
- 1 tablespoon lime juice

- Pinch of cayenne pepper

- Pinch of salt

How To Prepare

- Blend the green crab and avocado

- Pour into a cup and add lime juice, cayenne pepper, and sodium.

- Stir well.

Benefits

- Apples are a full way to obtain antioxidants and help lower cholesterol levels, prevent malignancy cell department, and protects against diabetes and asthma.

- Avocados are a high source of nutritional vitamins, nutrients, and healthy extra fat. It helps to lessen fat, lowers coronary disease risk, and decreases aging.

- The lime helps to regulate the Digestive system. It can help with gastritis, heartburn, and constipation.

- Cayenne pepper helps to lose weight by boosting the metabolic process, it also prevents cardiovascular diseases.

www.ingramcontent.com/pod-product-compliance
Lightning Source LLC
Chambersburg PA
CBHW060401080526
44583CB00012B/424